GASTRIC BYPASS

MEAL PLANS

&

Cookbook

------------------~----------------

A Comprehensive Pre & Post Gastric Bypass Surgery Meal Plans, Diet Guide & Cookbook

------------------~----------------

ALSO INCLUDES: MOST CRITICAL PRE AND POST SURGERY DIET GUIDELINES

BY

MONIKA SHAH

COPYRIGHT © 2016

A Message for Readers!

Get your System Right with Right Diet & Meals

This book has been specifically designed and written for people who are either planning for, or have already undergone the Gastric Bypass surgery for weight loss. This book will help you understand the various aspects of Gastric Bypass surgery and guide you through both Pre and Post-operative phases.

Let's take a closer look on what this book has to offer:

- **The Gastric Bypass Surgery Guide**: This part of the book educates you not only about the Gastric Bypass surgery itself but also its risks, health benefits, expected changes in your body and life, and the processes and general procedures that hospitals follow before, during and after the Gastric Bypass Surgery. This section is important for people who are planning to undergo the Gastric Bypass surgery in near future.

- **The Gastric Bypass Meal Plans and Diet Guide:** This part of the book educates you in detail about the pre and post-operative diet stages. You will explore the detailed pre and post-surgery dietary information that one should follow to sail through the healing period of weight loss surgery. For each of these diet stages, book will unfold the real goals, guidelines, diet control measures and foods to eat and avoid from various food groups in detail.

- **The Gastric Bypass Surgery Cookbook:** The cookbook has some really nice, healthy and homemade recipes which are designed especially for people who have undergone the Gastric Bypass surgery. The recipes in the book have been designed using very simple ingredients that people use in their kitchen every day or can find in the grocery stores very easily. Each recipe comes with the clear set of ingredients and instructions along with the accurate serving sizes.

Apart from the above mentioned sections, the book also covers some very important strategies that one may require to deal with post-surgery problems. It will also educate you about the various dietary supplements that one need post-surgery to supply the necessary nutrients to the body.

CONTENTS

UNDERSTANDING THE GASTRIC BYPASS SURGERY   **1**

THE CRITERIA   1
TYPES OF WEIGHT LOSS SURGERIES   2
     Sleeve Gastrectomy   3
     Laparoscopic Adjustable Gastric Banding   3
     Duodenal Switch with Biliopancreatic Diversion   3
     Roux-en-Y Gastric Bypass   4

RISKS ASSOCIATED WITH WEIGHT LOSS SURGERIES   **5**

SLEEVE GASTRECTOMY   5
LAPAROSCOPIC ADJUSTABLE GASTRIC BANDING   6
DUODENAL SWITCH WITH BILIOPANCREATIC DIVERSION   8
ROUX-EN-Y GASTRIC BYPASS   9

THE CHANGES IN YOUR BODY AND LIFE   **11**

ANATOMICAL CHANGES   11
HORMONAL ALTERATIONS   12
FAT LOSS   13
CO-EXISTING ILLNESSES   13
LONGEVITY   14
QUALITY OF LIFE   14

GENERAL HOSPITAL PROCEDURES, COSTS AND PROCESSES   **15**

PRE-GASTRIC BYPASS SURGERY DIET AND GUIDELINES   **19**

CRITICAL POST GASTRIC BYPASS SURGERY GUIDELINES   **23**

GUIDELINES FOR EATING   23
GUIDELINES FOR LIQUIDS   25
VARIOUS OTHER GUIDELINES   25

POST-SURGERY: MEAL PLANS, DIET GUIDELINES & RECIPES   **27**

POST-OPERATIVE DIET IN HOSPITAL   27
     Day 0 – The Day of Surgery   27
     Day 1 – The Day after Surgery   27

STAGE 1: WATER 28
 Goals and Duration 29
 Diet Guidelines 29
 Meal Suggestions 29
 Recipes: Stage 1 30

STAGE 2: SUGAR FREE CLEAR LIQUIDS 44
 Goals and Duration 45
 Diet Guidelines 45
 Meal Suggestions 46
 Recipes: Stage 2 47

STAGE 3: PUREED FOODS 61
 Goals and Duration 61
 Diet Guidelines 62
 Meal Suggestions 62
 Sample Menu 63
 Recipes: Stage 3 64

STAGE 4: SEMI-SOFT FOODS 75
 Goals and Duration 75
 Diet Guidelines 75
 Meal Suggestions 77
 Sample Menu 78
 Recipes: Stage 4 79

STAGE 5: REGULAR DIET 84
 Goals and Duration 84
 Diet Guidelines 85
 Meal Suggestions 86
 Sample Menu 87
 Recipes: Stage 5 88

DEALING WITH POST SURGERY PROBLEMS **117**

SUPPLEMENTS SUGGESTIONS **125**

WRAPPING UP! **129**

RECIPES INDEX **131**

Copyright Notes & Disclaimer

This Page Has Been Left Blank Intentionally.

Chapter 1

Understanding the Gastric Bypass Surgery

Probably, you have attempted all kinds of dietary and exercise regimens over the years, but failed to control your obesity. It could also be that your success, if any, was short-lived in nature. If you belong to the clinically obese category, it means that you have a chronic disease. Non-surgical treatment is not going to work for you. You will have to give serious thought to surgical procedures.

The Criteria

At the outset, your body mass index (BMI) must show a reading of 40 or more. The numerical figure is an indication of how much of excess fat has accumulated in your body. It is calculated in alignment with your height (feet and inches) and existing weight (pounds). This is because the amount of fat present in your body should be in proportion to your height and weight; it should not be in excess. Regardless of whether you are male or female, if your BMI is less than 18.5, you are in luck! Your weight is normal. You are overweight if the reading shows up as between 18.5 and 24.9. Anything beyond this number may be considered as 'obese.'

Since you are prone towards obesity, you cannot be expected to have a great quality of life. Despite trying out traditional weight loss programs on your own, as well as participating in closely supervised healthcare programs, you may have been unable to control your increasing girth. The doctor will wish to record every single detail.

The surgeon will want to know if you have a pre-existing medical or psychological condition, which can interfere with the overall benefits of gastric bypass surgery. If you are at great risk, you will not be allowed to have the operation.

However, if you have a co-morbid or medical condition that may be benefitted through weight loss, the doctor will advise you to go ahead with the surgery. To illustrate, you may have asthma, sleep apnea and other respiratory problems, issues with your cardiovascular system, arthritis, gastro-esophageal reflux disease (GERD), diabetes, or high levels of cholesterol in your blood.

You must be aware that only an adult can undergo this surgery. Therefore, you must be 18 years old, or even older. Then again, you must promise to adhere to the follow-up schedule, even if it goes on for a long time. Above all, you must be willing to go along with the surgeon's advice regarding post-operative lifestyle and dietary changes.

Types of Weight Loss Surgeries

Gastric bypass surgeries may be restrictive or malabsorptive in nature. The former ensures that the stomach shrinks in size, thereby losing the ability to hold as large amounts of food within it as prior to surgery. Naturally, when you eat less, your weight reduces. The latter, on the other hand, bypasses a portion of the smaller intestine, thereby preventing absorption of a large number of nutrients or calories. However, surgeons provide you with a smaller stomach too. Pure malabsorptive surgery can lead to unpleasant side effects.

Sleeve Gastrectomy

In this kind of restrictive surgery, the Bariatric surgeon will separate a small section of your stomach and remove it from your body. The portion left behind is given the approximate shape of a tube. Apart from the fact that your 'revised' stomach will not be able to contain much food, the surgery will also, reduce the production of ghrelin (appetite-regulating hormone).

Laparoscopic Adjustable Gastric Banding

This restrictive procedure involves fixing a band with an inflatable balloon around the upper region of your stomach. The balloon is akin to a pouch with a narrow opening, which leads to the lower portion of your stomach. Next, the surgeon will place a port possessing a tube, under the skin of your abdomen. The tube acts as the connection between the band and the port. You will be able to deflate or inflate the balloon by removing or injecting fluid through this port. Thus, your gastric band may be adjusted according to will.

Duodenal Switch with Biliopancreatic Diversion

This malabsorptive surgery begins with the removal of a large portion of your stomach. What is left behind is the stomach valve responsible for sending food to the small intestine, as well as the duodenum (first part of small intestine). The Bariatric surgeon will close off the middle part of your small intestine. Thus, it becomes possible to connect the duodenum and the last part of the small intestine directly, thereby creating the duodenal switch.

The Biliopancreatic diversion is created by re-connecting the separated middle section to the last section of the small intestine. This permits pancreatic and bile juices to flow into this region.

Roux-en-Y Gastric Bypass

This malabsorptive surgery comprises of the creation of a small pouch on the top of your stomach. All the food that you consume will enter this pouch only, and go nowhere else. However, digestive juices will continue to be made in your main stomach region. The surgeon will ensure that the portions of the small intestine present below the main stomach and attached to it, respectively, are cut and attached to the new pouch, as well as to one another.

Chapter 2

Risks Associated with Weight Loss Surgeries

Do not be under the impression that a surgical process is the ultimate cure for something chronic. Even a tried-and-proven method may be associated with some complications. The intention is not to frighten you. You are merely being advised to acquire clarity about any operation that you wish to undergo.

Sleeve Gastrectomy

Sleeve Gastrectomy is a relatively new procedure in comparison to the others. Here are some of the risks associated with this type of surgery.

- It is possible that the sleeve (tube) become dilated over the years, preventing sufficient weight loss.

- However, the biggest risk associated with this procedure is leakage. If this happens, you might require a second surgery, along with the placement of a feeding tube and a drainage tube. The tubes are temporary.

- Persistent leaks may lead to the formation of wounds or abscesses, thereby prompting a lengthy stay at the hospital.

- Wounds and infections may be treated with powerful antibiotics, but there is always the possibility of further complications.

- Then again, if you are prone towards heavy bleeding after the operation, you may require a blood transfusion.

- A careless surgeon may cause damage to the organs close to the operation site. If this should happen, you will require additional operative procedures.

- Although rare, it is possible that your 'revised' gut is unable to tolerate sufficient amounts of food. You will have to go in for total parenteral nutrition (TPN) then, that is, fed via intravenous methods.

- You may find a few blood clots accumulating in legs and traveling to your lungs. It happens rarely, but can prove fatal.

- Stay away from this procedure if you suffer from frequent heartburn.

Laparoscopic Adjustable Gastric Banding

Laparoscopic Adjustable Gastric Banding offers the following risks.

- You need not worry too much if you should experience diarrhea, constipation, regurgitation, acid reflux, or nausea, after the operation. You will be all right soon. Rush to the Emergency Room only if abdominal pain persists for a long time, such as beyond three hours.

- Leakage is an issue with this kind of surgery too; your Band may begin to leak. You may require a repeat operation.

- It is possible for the new implant to migrate and cause complications. This refers to displacement of the port, band erosion, or the band slipping from its place.

- Sometimes, the port becomes detached from the tubing, leading to all kinds of complications.

- Of course, like with any other surgical procedure, the site of the operation may become infected. Similarly, your stomach or esophagus may experience inflammation too. Antibiotics should help.

- It is quite possible for your esophagus to go into a spasm after the operation. However, this is not commonly witnessed.

- If you suffer from gastro-esophageal reflux disease (GERD), please avoid this type of surgery.

Duodenal Switch with Biliopancreatic Diversion

Duodenal Switch with Biliopancreatic Diversion also carries the same risks of infection along the staple line, leakage into the abdomen, and formation of blood clots in the legs and lungs. Apart from these, there are some specific long-term and short-term risks too.

- You might suffer from something known as the Dumping Syndrome, caused by an inability to tolerate processed sugars or highly refined and high-calorie foodstuffs. As soon as you consume sweet-tasting stuff, you experience nausea, cramping, sweating, extreme fatigue, dizziness or lightheadedness and heart palpitations. Explosive diarrhea can weaken you to such an extent that you have to lie down for some time.

- It is also possible to become a victim of frequent diarrhea and foul smelling stools, because your gut finds it difficult to absorb vitamins, protein, fats, iron and calcium.

- It follows that you will experience nutritional deficiency, as you become habituated to eating lesser and lesser food. You may have to consume vitamin supplements throughout your life.

- When you are nutritionally deficient, your bones become weak. Thus, you are at high risk for osteoporosis.

Roux-en-Y Gastric Bypass

Roux-en-Y Gastric Bypass tends to cause death in one amongst 200 patients (0.5% risk). Therefore, you should discuss this elective procedure thoroughly with your Bariatric surgeon before you proceed with it.

- Apart from the possibility of infection at the site of surgery, formation of blood clots, vitamin deficiency or leakage into the abdominal cavity, you may even become anemic or develop osteoporosis.

- Sometimes, your gallbladder is also removed during the surgical process. In case, it is not, gallstones may accumulate within it. The doctor will advise the consumption of preventive medications.

- If you do not drink sufficient water, you might get kidney stones.

- It is possible for your intestine to twist around itself, thereby causing hernia.

- You may require a second operation to resolve issues related to the newly created pouch or strictures (connections become too narrow).

- Frequent failure to adhere to changes in diet or lifestyle, may lead to weight gain instead of weight loss.

This Page Has Been Left Blank Intentionally.

Chapter 3

The Changes in Your Body and Life

The risks outlined above are just possibilities, dependent upon your individual constitution. They are not confirmed outcomes for every single patient who opts for Gastric Bypass surgery. Therefore, give importance to the advice of reputed organizations like the U.S. National Institutes of Health. Even they suggest that the only option left for you is to go in for Bariatric surgery, especially if you wish to maintain your weight loss for a long time to come.

Anatomical Changes

On its own, obesity may not prove to be such a tremendous problem, except for making you look ungainly and preposterous. Unfortunately, it invites life-threatening conditions to intrude into your life. You have to find a way to enhance fat metabolism and ensure that the right nutrients reach your bodily cells. Gastric Bypass surgery is the right tool for this process. This operation brings about specific changes in the anatomy of your gastrointestinal tract, as outlined in an earlier chapter.

These changes influence the production of intestinal hormones, such that you feel satiated even with small quantities of food. Feelings of hunger, as well as your regular appetite are reduced significantly. It follows that you will no longer go in for frequent bouts of eating. If combined with nutritive meals, regular exercise and modification in behavior, the operation can prove to be highly rewarding.

Hormonal Alterations

Now, the hormonal changes that occur through normal dietary weight loss and those that are induced via surgery, differ. For instance, when you go in for specific nutrition programs, you expect some changes in body composition to take place, along with a predicted weight loss. It does happen, as you want it to. However, you may not be aware that your energy expenditure is being greatly reduced too, leaving you feeling tired and listless. This is because dietary programs do not focus much on balanced meals, but on reduction of calories in whichever way possible. Therefore, it is quite possible that the imbalance induces you to feel hungrier and eat more, thereby leading to weight regain.

Bariatric surgery, on the other hand, focuses on energy expenditure, that is, burning a larger amount of calories. The hormonal changes induced by this operation aid in maintaining or increasing the expenditure of energy. You may rest assured that you will not lose too much of energy, for the expenditure is proportionate to the changes in your body size. Since energy balance is initiated and maintained, your surgery-induced weight loss is bound to sustain for a long time.

Fat Loss

Obviously, your metabolic processes are at fault, since you tend to put on weight so easily. When you find your body coming back to a normal size after surgery, you tend to engage in all kinds of physical activities. In fact, you may even develop a fancy for vigorous outdoor sports, like swimming, walking, hiking, biking, and so on. It is to be expected that as you toil and sweat, your body begins to burn the excess fat accumulated in varied regions.

In turn, you will feel less stressed and begin to develop a more positive attitude towards life in general. The entire credit may be attributed to the reduction in insulin (helps to regulate glucose levels in your bloodstream) secretions and cortisol (causes stress) secretions. Combined with other factors, these hormones serve to decrease the uptake and storage of excess fat into your body.

Experts suggest that you should be able to maintain greater than 50% or even more of your excess weight loss after Bariatric surgery. Just about 10% of patients fail to do so, maybe due to additional complications.

Co-existing Illnesses

You may be having co-morbid diseases caused by obesity, and even worsened in alignment with your expanding girth. Such co-morbidities may become acute, chronic, or life threatening, if suitable measures are not undertaken. To illustrate, weight loss can bring about drastic improvement even in a person suffering from Type II Diabetes Mellitus, as evinced by review of literature related to 621 scientific studies.

According to the American Society for Metabolic and Bariatric Surgery, around 85% of the 135,247 diabetes-afflicted volunteers, who participated in these studies, exhibited wonderful improvement after Gastric Bypass surgeries. Many people even experienced remission of diabetic disease. Admittedly, weight loss does pay.

Longevity

Who does not wish to live longer? Gastric Bypass surgery tends to lower the risk of death, especially when you are suffering from a dangerous ailment. True, Bariatric operations carry their own risks, but they offer great benefits too. Do follow the surgeon's post-operative instructions carefully, and reduce your mortality rate.

Quality of Life

You are bound to discover positive changes in areas like disability, mobility, sexual function, work, unemployment, social interactions, self-esteem, mental health, etc., after your Bariatric surgery. Naturally, your quality of life should improve to a great deal.

Chapter 4

General Hospital Procedures, Costs and Processes

You cannot just walk into a Bariatric clinic and admit yourself as a patient. You will have to submit to an in-depth evaluation conducted by experienced professionals first. They are part of a multidisciplinary team, which takes into account your existing physical condition, mental status, nutritional habits and lifestyle, before selecting or rejecting you for surgery.

Some institutes set up general seminars, in order to disseminate information about Bariatric surgery. Such informative sessions help you to prepare yourself better for what might lie ahead, as well as, create a list of questions that you might like answered by the surgeon concerned.

Regardless of whether you attend such a seminar or not, you will have to take the help of your primary care provider for setting up an appointment with a Bariatric surgeon. After the appointment is fixed, you may have to fill up certain documents with details about your personal history, past medical history, current medications, allergies, etc. You will have to submit them to the Bariatric surgeon during the initial consultation.

After going through these forms during the first consultation, the Bariatric surgeon may request further information about your existing co-morbidities. Do not leave out any details of your past or present experiences. Rest assured; there will be no breach of confidentiality. You would not like to invite further complications in your life by leaving out vital information, would you?

Once the assessment is complete and the surgeon has clarified all your doubts, he/she will provide information about the kind of Gastric Bypass procedure that is most suitable for you. Yes, even the risks associated with it will be discussed. Finally, you will be requested to undergo certain tests, such as complete blood picture, electrocardiogram to discover the condition of your heart, screening for diabetes, etc. In case, you suffer from sleep apnea, you will have to undergo a sleep study.

Mere physical and laboratory evaluations will not suffice to categorize you as a suitable patient for Gastric Bypass surgery. You will need to undergo a psychological assessment too. It is imperative that the psychologist comprehend how your choices and quality of life have been affected by your "weighty" problems. After all, you have to be willing to make major changes in your life after the surgery. You cannot afford to be emotionally weak. In fact, the counselor may even advise you to take certain medications to improve your mental status, as well as make appointments for regular psychotherapy sessions, if the situation warrants it.

Does the dietitian have a role to play in this scenario? Yes, he/she definitely has! In fact, you will have to set up several sessions with this well-qualified and well-trained expert, prior to your surgery. Provide her with every single detail about your past dietary habits and your attempts at losing excess weight. Armed with this information, he/she will be able to provide guidance regarding the new eating habits that have to be adopted after Bariatric surgery. If you are serious about weight loss, you will need to have tips about the diet regimen to be followed at home, what foodstuffs to choose when you eat out, how your choices influence your stress levels and moods, etc.

When the results of all your tests and evaluations have been submitted to the Bariatric surgeon, he/she will invite you for a final consult. The details of the surgery under question and the complications associated with it will also be discussed once again. If everything proves satisfactory, the doctor will request your approval for the surgery. Do not worry; you will be granted some time to think everything over and get back at your convenience.

Every hospital has its rules and regulations, as well as its unique payment structure. Some of the staff may be deemed as visiting staff; they demand their own fees. Therefore, whether you do so during the initial consult or final meeting, do not forget to request details about the costs associated with the surgery, hospital stay, post-operative care, etc. Note that you are going in for elective (not compulsory) surgery, not something that is imperative to improve your health.

Your insurance company may not be willing to finance you 100%; you will have to share the expenses. Take the assistance of the administrative staff at the concerned clinic for dealing with your insurance coverage, as well as requesting pre-authorization for your surgical procedure. They will even supply supporting documents with your insurance forms, to strengthen your case. On your part, you have to be patient. Some insurance companies provide approval rapidly, while others take over a month to do so.

When everything has been resolved to satisfaction, you may fix a date for your surgery. A week before that, you will have to submit to a thorough physical examination and pre-admission testing.

This Page Has Been Left Blank Intentionally.

Chapter 5

Pre-Gastric Bypass Surgery Diet and Guidelines

Two weeks prior to your surgery, the dietitian will advise you to adhere to a diet that is low in fats and carbohydrates. As a result, the liver will be forced to release the glycogen (form of sugar) stored within it, for your organ systems to function properly. As the glycogen stores continue to deplete, your liver will soften and shrink in size.

Your Bariatric surgeon will appreciate this phenomenon, especially if he/she is going in for laparoscopic (keyhole) surgery and not open surgery. The liver has to be lifted and shifted aside for him/her to gain access to your stomach. It would be difficult if the liver were heavy, immobile and filled with excess fat. Note that most Bariatric surgeons prefer to avoid open surgery, since it results in a large abdominal scar, a lengthier recovery period and enhanced risks.

Then again, it is imperative that you lose at least 10 to 15 pounds before surgery. In case, your BMI is over 55, you will need to reduce at least 10% of your total body weight.

The Two-week Diet

You have to stay off any kind of solid food for a fortnight. It is important that your body receive at least 800 to 1000 calories each day via fluids. Please stick to clear liquids only, mainly water.

A protein shake should serve as a meal replacement. Use skimmed milk or ice-cold water along with four to six ounces or a scoop of protein powder, for each shake. Use a blender to mix everything properly. Consume these shakes thrice a day.

Initially, as your body tries to adjust to this diet, you may experience headaches and irritation. Regardless, please do not go in for any kind of herbal medications or non-steroidal anti-inflammatory drugs (NSAIDs) at this time. You have no idea of how your digestive system will react to these herbs, while you are off solid food. As for NSAIDs, they tend to cause excessive bleeding, especially during the post-operative period.

In case, you are on specific medications for particular health conditions, please consult with your PCP beforehand. The altered shape of your stomach caused by Gastric Bypass surgery may not prove suitable to hold large pills. Your PCP will have to ensure that you take medicines in a chewable, liquid, or crushed form. Time-released drugs may not work as effectively if they are crushed. Request your PCP to provide alternatives and give guidance on how to adjust the medications with your new diet pre-operatively and post-operatively. Do not stop taking them on your own. If you are a diabetic, ensure that your blood sugar levels remain stable throughout the two weeks.

Last 24-hour Diet

You are requested to stay on a pure and clear liquid diet. Stop all protein shakes. You may have water, tea, jello, broth and ginger ale.

The Night before Surgery

Avoid all liquids and solids. In fact, you cannot have anything to eat or drink by mouth. Your stomach must be empty at the time of the operation.

This Page Has Been Left Blank Intentionally.

Chapter 6

Critical Post Gastric Bypass Surgery Guidelines

The dietary regimen that you follow post-op, will be different from the one that you followed prior to your opting for Gastric Bypass surgery.

Guidelines for Eating

You may be surprised to discover a sense of fullness even after eating a small meal. This is because the size of your stomach has reduced and the length of your small intestine or small bowel has shortened. During the first few days after the operation, the surgeon will advise you to restrict both, the volume and consistency of food, since your internal wounds must heal.

- You must get into the habit of eating very slowly. If you are keen to gobble up everything on your plate as fast as possible, do not be surprised when you throw up, or feel nauseous. This happens when you consume a very small meal. Therefore, pace your meal, such that you take at least 30 minutes to eat it.

- Chew every piece of food until it acquires a liquid consistency. Then, swallow it. It takes time and practice to master the art of chewing well. Large chunks of food can block the outlets in your revised alimentary tract.

- Please do not be greedy. Adhere to the amounts suggested for every meal, if you do not wish to vomit or feel nauseous. It is possible to rupture your stomach or cause it to expand through careless eating. Above all, you may begin to regain weight.

- You may experience Dumping syndrome, if you insist on gorging on ice creams, soda, puddings, cakes, cookies, pies, chocolates, etc. As these sugary or high-calorie foods rush from the stomach to the small intestine, you may begin to exhibit symptoms of weakness, cramping, nausea, sweating, rapid heart rate, a feeling of uncomfortable fullness and explosive diarrhea. Continue with your unhealthy habits, and you will find your body being deprived of essential nutrients. Maintaining weight loss will become problematic.

- Find out if your stomach can still feel compatible with high-fiber foods, red meat, milk, etc. You will know when you experience diarrhea, discomfort or nausea. If the dietitian permits you to experiment with substitutes or new foods, eat them in minimal amounts only. Consume only one new food at a time. If you cannot digest it properly, give yourself a gap of one week, and try again. If you still cannot tolerate it, eliminate it from your diet.

- Ensure that you purchase all the recommended minerals and vitamins prior to surgery, as well as consume them regularly in alignment with your prescription.

Guidelines for Liquids

- Similar to consumption of solid foods, even liquids must be drunk very slowly. Do remember that they have to undergo digestion too.

- Never combine water or drinks with meals. With regard to water, please consume it half-an-hour or an hour before a meal. Alternatively, you may wait for an hour or so after your meal, before drinking water. Otherwise, you are bound to experience nausea and vomiting. Your stomach may expand, and even rupture.

- This does not mean that you have to avoid liquids, or keep them to a minimum. Please consume loads of fluids. You need them to keep your body well hydrated. You can even become dehydrated through frequent bouts of diarrhea or vomiting. Therefore, ensure that you consume at least three to four ounces of water between meals. You may even go in for acceptable low-calorie beverages.

Various Other Guidelines

Three days of hospitalization should suffice after your Gastric Bypass operation. It is possible that you will develop life-threatening blood clots. In order to prevent this, your surgeon will advise you not to keep lying down in bed, but to sit in a chair for as long as possible. Additionally, even if you are in pain, you will be forced to walk around, albeit with assistance. This is to ensure healthy blood circulation.

Since the newly created connections in your digestive system need time to heal, you will not be permitted to eat or drink anything on the day of the surgery. The next day, you may be permitted to take sips of water. Thereafter, you will be advised on the various phases of a pre-determined dietary regimen that you must follow for healthy recovery and maintenance of weight loss.

If your condition is good, you will be discharged after three days. Please adhere to the follow-up schedule charted out for you. The first follow-up will be a couple of weeks after your surgery. In case, you experience frequent vomiting, nausea, fever, chills, or worsening pain in the first two weeks, please request an emergency consultation with your Bariatric surgeon. Do the same if your incisions show signs of painful inflammation.

Chapter 7

Post-Surgery: Meal Plans, Diet Guidelines & Recipes

Post-Operative Diet in Hospital

Day 0 – The Day of Surgery

You will not be permitted to take anything by mouth on this day. In simple words, you will not be allowed to ingest any kind of foodstuffs, beverages or medications. Your surgical wounds have to heal. Your "new" stomach will not be able to adjust to the entry of food so soon.

Day 1 – The Day after Surgery

Your stomach is now in a position to tolerate fluids, but not solid food. You may consume 30 cc (one ounce) of water every hour, throughout the day. However, do not gulp down the contents in your glass at one go. Just sip slowly, as slowly as possible. No, you may not use a straw to drink water. Ice chips are not allowed either.

The water should be neither too warm nor too cold. Drink it at room temperature. Note that your gut will not be able to tolerate liquids having extreme temperatures for quite some time. It would be best to be careful for the first three months at least.

You will be observed throughout the day. If you do not experience nausea or vomiting, you may advance to the next phase of your diet.

Stage 1: Water

On the second day following your operation, you will be placed on a sugar-free, clear-liquid diet. You may be at risk for nausea and vomiting as your stomach remains empty, while trying to cope with the trauma of Bariatric surgery. Regardless, your body requires nourishment. Therefore, fill your stomach with fluids and experience that sense of fullness.

It is also necessary to keep your body well hydrated, in order to avoid complications like dehydration and constipation. Fluids also help to flush out harmful waste products.

Acceptable liquids include:

- Pure water
- Flavored water (non-carbonated)
- Sugar-free popsicles (around 20 calories, that is, two per day)
- Sugar-free jello
- Decaffeinated coffee or tea
- Clear beef broth or bouillon
- Chicken broth
- Gelatin,
- Two cups of fruit juices (cranberry, apple or grape) per day
- Ice chips and low-calorie sports drinks (non-carbonated)

Goals and Duration

You will have to adhere to this diet for one week.

Your goal with regard to fluids is to reach six cups or 48 ounces (use a one-ounce medicine cup) of nutrient-enriched, acceptable liquids, each day.

Diet Guidelines

Please sip every kind of fluid as slowly as possible. Do not force yourself to finish a drink if you experience abdominal discomfort or stomach fullness. Never take liquids half-an-hour before a solid meal or for 60 minutes after it. Maintain a daily journal of your eating and drinking habits.

Meal Suggestions

Breakfast may comprise of a one-half cup of low-sodium broth or one-half cup of sugar-free jello. Maintain the same menu for lunch and dinner.

Alternatively, your breakfast may include apple juice (2 tablespoons) along with chicken broth and diet gelatin (three tablespoons each). For lunch, substitute cranberry juice and beef broth for apple juice and chicken broth. At dinner, let your choice of fruit juice be grape juice.

Recipes: Stage 1

A MESSAGE FOR READERS

You must adjust the quantity of ingredients based on the servings you are preparing. The current quantities are generic and written to just give you an idea on which ingredient should be added in more quantity and which one in less quantity.

FLAVORED WATER RECIPES

THE STRAWBERRY WATER

Serving Size: 2-3 tablespoons

Ingredients

4-6 strawberries, hulled and quartered
1/2 lemon, sliced
Small handful of basil, scrunched
1 liter ice and cold filtered water

Directions

1. Fill your juice pitcher to the top with ice and fruit.
2. Slightly scrunch up the basil so it releases its flavour.
3. Cover with cold filtered water.
4. Strain well and serve.

THE WATERMELON WATER

Serving Size: 2-3 tablespoons

Ingredients

2 slices of watermelon cut into thirds or quarters
Small handful of basil, scrunched
1 liter ice and cold filtered water

Directions

1. Fill your juice pitcher to the top with ice and fruit.
2. Slightly scrunch up the basil so it releases its flavour.
3. Cover with cold filtered water.
4. Strain well and serve.

THE ORANGE & BLUEBERRY WATER

Serving Size: 2-3 tablespoons

Ingredients

6 cups water
2 mandarin oranges cut into wedges
A handful of blueberries
Ice

Directions

1. Combine all ingredients in a pitcher and put in the fridge for 2 to 24 hours in order to allow the water to infuse.
2. You can also squeeze in the juice of one mandarin orange and muddle the blueberries to intensify flavour a bit.
3. Strain really well and serve.

THE ROSEMARY & GRAPEFRUIT WATER

Serving Size: 2-3 tablespoons

Ingredients

1/2 grapefruit
Several sprigs of Rosemary
Water
Ice

Directions

1. Add ingredients to the bottom of a pitcher.
2. Cover with water.
3. Let sit overnight.
4. Strain well and serve.

THE MANGO & GINGER WATER

Serving Size: 2-3 tablespoons

Ingredients

1 inch Ginger Root, peeled and sliced
1 cup Frozen or Fresh Mango
3 cups of ice
Water

Directions

1. Start by peeling the ginger. Only peel the part that you will be using. Slice the ginger into 3 to 4 coin sized slices. You want them about the size and thickness of the coin.
2. Drop the peeled and sliced ginger into your pitcher and add in the mango.
3. Top with 3 cups of ice and then add water.
4. Place in your fridge for 1 to 3 hours.
5. Strain well and serve.

THE MELON MIX WATER

Serving Size: 2-3 tablespoons

Ingredients

1 cup cantaloupe pieces
1 cup watermelon pieces
1 cup honeydew pieces
2 quarts filtered or spring water

Directions

1. Add your melons to a 64-ounce Mason jar or pitcher.
2. Pour the water over top and chill. Serve over ice.
3. Place in your fridge for 1 to 3 hours.
4. Strain well and serve.

CLEAR BROTH RECIPES

SIMPLE CLEAR BEEF BONE BROTH

Serving Size: 2-3 tablespoons

Ingredients

Beef bones with marrow
Water to cover bones
3 tbsp. apple cider vinegar
2 Bay Leaves
Sea Salt and Ground Black Pepper
Vegetables of choice

Directions

1. Place all ingredients in crockpot.
2. Add in water until bones are covered.
3. Turn setting to high and let simmer for 48 hours
4. Skim the fat off, strain well and serve.

EASY CLEAR BEEF BONE BROTH - VERSION 2

Serving Size: 2-3 tablespoons

Ingredients

2 pounds of beef bones
2 tablespoons of vinegar
3 quarts of water
1 peeled onion
1 carrot
2 celery stalks
1 garlic clove
A pinch of sea salt and ground black pepper for taste

Directions

1. Roast the raw beef bones for about 30 to 45 minutes at 350 degrees for the best flavour.
2. Add bones to crock pot or stove-top pot.
3. Add vegetables.
4. Cover the bones and vegetables with water until the beef bones are completely covered and the water level is about one inch above the bones.
5. Add vinegar.
6. Turn crock pot on low.
7. Watch the broth in the first few hours and skim off any "scum" that may rise to the top.
8. Stew your bones for about 24 hours.
9. Skim the fat off, strain really well and serve.

SIMPLE CLEAR CHICKEN BONE BROTH

Serving Size: 2-3 tablespoons

Ingredients

Chicken necks and feet
Water to cover
3 tbsp. apple cider vinegar
Sea Salt and Ground Black Pepper
2 Bay Leaves
Garlic cloves
Vegetables of choice

Directions

1. Place all ingredients into stock pot and add enough water until chicken is submerged.
2. Turn setting to high until it boils, then turn to low and simmer for 24 hours.
3. Skim the fat off, strain really well and serve.

THE VEGETABLE BROTH

Serving Size: 2-3 tablespoons

Ingredients

2 carrots
1 red onion
1 fennel
3 celery stalks
6 sprigs of flat-leaf parsley
6 sprigs of fresh thyme
3 slices of fresh ginger
4 cloves of garlic
10-20 coriander seeds
8-10 black peppercorns
1 Turkish bay leaf
1 tbsp. sea salt
10 cups of water

Directions

1. Wash and cut your vegetables into big chunks and place in a large saucepan or stock pot.
2. Add herbs, spices and cold water.
3. Pass through a fine mesh strainer.
4. At this point, if you prefer a richer broth, you can reduce the vegetable broth by cooking it further to get a more concentrated flavour. If not, proceed with storing.
5. Let the stock cool to room temperature. Place the amount of stock you intend to use immediately (up to three days) in a glass jar with a lid and place it in your refrigerator.
6. For the remaining, place 1 cup portions in freezer bags or

pour the vegetable broth in ice cube trays and freeze. If you're freezing the vegetable broth in ice cube trays, once frozen, make sure to place the cubes in an air-tight container.

Stage 2: Sugar Free Clear Liquids

Your stomach is apt to remain swollen and uncooperative for a few weeks following your Gastric Bypass surgery. Regardless, adhere to a sensible diet as much as possible, without depriving yourself of essential nutrients.

You may include various sugar-free liquids in your diet, such as:

- Gelatin
- Jello
- Beverages
- Nutritional supplements
- Popsicles (2 each day)
- Kool Aid
- Custard mix
- Pulp-free fruit juices (8 ounces each day or 4 ounces per serving)
- Applesauce
- Pudding mix
- Cream of rice/wheat cereal and Gatorade (just 8 ounces each day)

You may also consume:

- Tomato juice (strained)
- Low-fat cream soups
- Crystal light
- Plain yoghurt
- Reduced-calorie and smooth yoghurt
- Herbal tea
- Decaffeinated flat diet soda
- Non-fat (1%) milk

- Infant strained fruits
- Plain soy milk (of lactaid milk)
- Dry milk powder (non-fat)
- Soy/whey protein powder (as protein shakes)
- Bottled water (non-carbonated and non-flavored).

Goals and Duration

This diet has to continue for a couple of weeks after your surgery, that is, until your first follow-up.

As for goals, your body requires around 70 g of protein each day. Whatever kind of product you opt for, the label displays the approximate quantity per serving. Use this information to help you calculate the quantity of your protein shake correctly.

Then again, you will have to consume four ounces of sugar-free, nutritional supplements around eight times a day (a drink every two hours).

Please add three chewable calcium carbonate plus vitamin D tablets (600 mg each), two chewable multivitamins (for adults) and vitamin B Complex to your new dietary regimen. Ingest each one with a meal, as this will promote healthy absorption.

Diet Guidelines

As suggested earlier, please eat and drink very, very slowly. In fact, it would be best to get into the habit of sipping leisurely. Yes, do take half-an-hour to consume any liquid.

Then again, do not use a straw at any cost. The straw tends to draw in air, which will reach your stomach eventually. As a result, you are bound to experience pain, pressure, bloating or excessive gas formation. Apart from abdominal discomfort, you may experience pain in the shoulder and chest region too.

You might schedule your liquids to stretch out over three-hour intervals. This should help you keep well hydrated throughout the day.

Liquids are not meant to be a part of your regular meals. They must be drunk at least half-an-hour before a meal, or an hour after the meal.

If you cannot tolerate plain milk, look for suitable substitutes.

Meal Suggestions

Have half-a-cup each of meal replacement (sugar free) and skimmed milk, along with half-a-scoop of protein powder. For lunch, you might try sugar-free and fat-free yoghurt (half-a-cup). Dinner might consist of strained, low-fat cream soup (half-a-cup). Drink plenty of liquids between meals.

Alternatively, you may opt for a breakfast comprising of cream of wheat and plain/smooth and reduced-calorie yoghurt (one-fourth cup each). Lunch may consist of strained soup and sugar-free pudding (one-fourth cup each). For dinner, try one-fourth cup each of reduced-calorie yoghurt and strained soup.

Recipes: Stage 2

A MESSAGE FOR READERS

You must adjust the quantity of ingredients based on the servings you are preparing. The current quantities are generic and written to just give you an idea on which ingredient should be added in more quantity and which one in less quantity.

HERBAL TEAS RECIPES

THE NERVE SOOTHER TEA

Serving Size: 2-3 tablespoons

Ingredients

1 tablespoon chamomile
1 tablespoon peppermint

Directions

1. Place the ingredients in equal proportion above into 8oz of fresh boiling water.
2. You may use a teaball or cloth teabag if you do not want to have to strain your tea prior to drinking.
3. Let it steep for 5 full minutes.
4. Remove the herbs, strain really well and enjoy.

THE BRAIN GAINER TEA

Serving Size: 2-3 tablespoons

Ingredients

1 teaspoon gingko
1 teaspoon ginseng (or you can use liquid concentrate – 1 little bottle)
1 teaspoon peppermint

Directions

1. Place the ingredients above into 16 oz. of fresh boiling water.
2. Place the lid on the pot.
3. Use a teaball or cloth teabag if you do not want to have to strain you tea prior to drinking.
4. Let it steep for 5-10 full minutes.
5. Strain well and serve.

THE GOOD MOOD TEA

Serving Size: 2-3 tablespoons

Ingredients

1 teaspoon st johns wort
1 teaspoon chamomile

Directions

1. Place the ingredients in equal proportion above into 8oz of fresh boiling water.
2. Use a teaball or cloth teabag if you do not want to have to strain you tea prior to drinking.
3. Put the lid on the pot.
4. Let it steep for 5 full minutes.
5. Sweeten with honey and serve.

LET'S FEEL LIGHT TEA

Serving Size: 2-3 tablespoons

Ingredients

1 tablespoon peppermint
Dash of rosemary
Dash of sage

Directions

1. Place the ingredients in above into 8oz of fresh boiling water.
2. Use a teaball or cloth teabag if you do not want to have to strain you tea prior to drinking.
3. Put the lid on the pot.
4. Let it steep for 5 full minutes.
5. Remove the herbs and enjoy.

VITAMIN C BOOSTER TEA

Serving Size: 2-3 tablespoons

Ingredients

1 tablespoon dried rose hips – crushed if you like
1 tablespoon dried berries, (strawberries, blueberries etc.)

Directions

1. Place the ingredients in above into 8oz of fresh boiling water.
2. Use a tea ball or cloth teabag if you do not want to have to strain you tea prior to drinking.
3. Put the lid on the pot.
4. Let it steep for 5 full minutes.
5. Remove the herbs and enjoy.

GINGER & PEPPERMINT HERBAL TEA

Serving Size: 2-3 tablespoons

Ingredients

1 inch ginger root, sliced
1 tablespoon peppermint

Directions

1. Place the ingredients in equal proportion above into 16 oz. of fresh boiling water.
2. Use a tea ball or cloth teabag if you do not want to have to strain you tea prior to drinking.
3. Let it steep for 5 full minutes.
4. Strain well and serve.

THE EARL GREY HERBAL TEA

Serving Size: 2-3 tablespoons

Ingredients

1 tablespoon bee balm
1 tablespoon bergamot

Directions

1. Place the ingredients in above into 16 oz. of fresh boiling water.
2. Use a tea ball or cloth teabag if you do not want to have to strain you tea prior to drinking.
3. Let it steep for 5 full minutes.
4. Remove the herbs and enjoy.
5. Sweeten with honey if you like.

STRAWBERRY & LEMON HERBAL TEA

Serving Size: 2-3 tablespoons

Ingredients

1 tablespoon dried strawberries
1 tablespoon lemon balm leaves, bruised

Directions

1. Place the ingredients in above into 16 oz. of fresh boiling water.
2. Use a tea ball or cloth teabag if you do not want to have to strain you tea prior to drinking.
3. Let it steep for 5 full minutes.
4. Remove the herbs and enjoy.
5. Sweeten with honey if you like.

LOW FAT SOUPS RECIPES

LOW-FAT CREAM OF MUSHROOM SOUP

Serving Size: 2-3 tablespoons to ¼ cup (Gradually increase after a few days)

Ingredients

1 tablespoon olive oil
3 leeks, chopped (white part only)
2 garlic cloves, minced
1/2 sweet onion, chopped
1 teaspoon crushed red pepper
Pinch kosher salt
Pinch fresh ground pepper
1 pound fresh mushrooms, chopped
1 tablespoon all-purpose flour
32 ounces beef, chicken, or vegetable stock
1 cup evaporated milk
1 tablespoon dried thyme

Directions

1. Heat oil in a large pot over medium heat.
2. Cook leeks, garlic, onions and red pepper, stirring frequently, for 5 minutes or until leeks are tender. Season with salt and pepper.
3. Add mushrooms and cook, stirring occasionally, for 5 minutes until tender.
4. Stir in flour, stock, milk and thyme. Cook for about 10 minutes, stirring occasionally. Let cool slightly.

5. In batches, pour soup into a blender or food processor and blend until creamy.
6. Reheat when ready to serve. Simmer, do not boil.

LOW-FAT CREAM OF ASPARAGUS

Serving Size: 2-3 tablespoons to ¼ cup (Gradually increase after a few days)

Ingredients

2 teaspoons olive oil
1-1/2 pounds asparagus, cut into 2-inch pieces
1 medium onion, chopped
1 celery stalk, chopped
2 leeks, chopped (white part only)
1 medium potato, peeled, cut into 1-inch pieces
3-1/2 cups fat-free reduced-sodium chicken or vegetable broth
1/2 cup fat-free sour cream

Directions

1. Heat oil in a large pot over medium heat.
2. Cook asparagus, onion, celery, leeks and potatoes, stirring occasionally, about 5 minutes.
3. Add broth and simmer 20 minutes or until vegetables are tender.
4. In batches, pour soup into a blender or food processor and blend until smooth.
5. Pour soup back into pot and stir in sour cream. Heat, stirring, until combined — do not boil.
6. Serve warm.

Stage 3: Pureed Foods

This is the third stage when your stomach is in a position to accept pureed foods. Acceptable foodstuffs in this stage include:

- Veggie cheese
- Cottage cheese (1%)
- Low-fat cheese (2 g fat per serving)
- Skimmed milk
- Sugar-free and low-fat yoghurt
- Eggs (only one yolk each day)
- Eggbeaters (whipping cream)
- Canned chicken
- Tuna fish (packed in water) and pureed/soft protein.

Fresh white fish like flounder, shrimp, scallops, Cod, sole and imitation crabmeat are extremely suitable too. You may also favor legumes like garbanzos or chickpeas, kidney beans and black beans. Another set of foods include soy products, tofu and BOCA burgers. As for meats, opt for low-fat varieties, or healthy ham and Turkey breast.

Goals and Duration

You will have to adhere to this diet for a period of three weeks.

By offering your digestive system more choices in the form of blended or pureed foodstuffs, you face a lower risk of falling prey to bouts of nausea or vomiting.

Diet Guidelines

You must remember to chew every piece of food to a liquid or paste-like consistency, prior to swallowing.

Ensure that protein-containing foods are ground to baby food consistency via a blender. Otherwise, your stomach and intestine may become blocked. This will result in tremendous abdominal pain, nausea or vomiting.

Proteins are marvelous for healing wounds and reducing muscle loss. Therefore, they should reach your stomach first.

Whatever you eat, eat very slowly with the aid of a baby spoon or a small saucer. **From handling just a couple of tablespoons in the beginning, you will gradually progress to half-a-cup or four ounces of food at every meal.**

If you are keen on experimenting with new foods, please tackle only one novel item at a time.

Continue the intake of mineral and vitamin supplements as suggested earlier.

The rules for liquid consumption remain the same always.

Meal Suggestions

Protein Suggestions: Low-carbohydrate or sugar-free Carnation Instant Breakfast, mashed tofu, Skimor (1%) milk (a couple of cups each day), low-calorie yoghurt, eggbeaters or scrambled eggs, blended chunky soups, strained cream soups, mashed beans (pinto, black or fat-free refried), ricotta cheese and low-fat cottage cheese. As for meats, you may go in for baby food meats, pureed lean beef, fish, lean pork, turkey or chicken.

Grains and Starches – Sweet potatoes, winter squash or mashed potatoes are healthy. Amongst hot cereals, you might try oatmeal, cream of wheat/rice, grits and Malt-o-Meal.

Fruits and Vegetables – Try mashed bananas, pureed fruits (apricots, peaches, pears, etc.), sugar-free and plain applesauce and pureed vegetables (beets, carrots, green beans, etc.).

Sample Menu

Partake of one-fourth cup each of mashed scrambled eggs and oatmeal at breakfast. Thirty minutes later, consume Carnation Instant Breakfast (half-a-cup). Thereafter, consume half-a-cup of calorie-free drink or water, every half-an-hour (three times). Repeat this procedure after lunch and dinner too.

For lunch, have one-fourth cup each of pureed peaches and mashed low-fat cottage cheese.

Dinner may be a combination of pureed chicken or baby food meat (one-fourth cup), pureed green beans (one-eighth cup) and applesauce (one-eighth cup). Substitute Carnation Instant Breakfast with half-a-cup of plain milk (1%) or skimmed milk.

Recipes: Stage 3

A MESSAGE FOR READERS

You must adjust the quantity of ingredients based on the servings you are preparing. The current quantities are generic and written to just give you an idea on which ingredient should be added in more quantity and which one in less quantity.

PUREED FOODS RECIPES

PUREED BLACK BEAN SOUP

Serving Size: 2-3 tablespoons to ½ cup (Gradually increase after a few days)

Ingredients

½ tablespoon of coconut or other healthy cooking oil
½ chopped onion
¼ teaspoon of chili powder
½ teaspoon of ground cumin
1 15-ounce can of black beans, rinsed
1 ½ cups of water
1/4 cup of low sodium mild salsa
1 teaspoon of lime juice
Dash of salt substitute and ground pepper

Directions

1. First, heat the oil in a large saucepan on medium heat. Add chopped onion and cook two or three minutes, until onion softens and becomes clear.
2. Add chilli powder, cumin and other spices and continue to cook for one minute longer.
3. Add the beans, salsa and water and bring mixture to a boil.
4. Reduce heat to simmer and leave for ten minutes; remove and stir in lime juice.
5. Transfer to a blender and puree before returning the mixture to the saucepan.
6. Serve the pureed bean soup garnished with low fat sour cream if desired.

PUREED CAULIFLOWER SOUP

Serving Size: 2-3 tablespoons to ½ cup (Gradually increase after a few days)

Ingredients

1 ¼ cups of low-sodium, low-fat chicken broth
½ head of cauliflower florets
Salt substitute and mild ground pepper for seasoning
½ teaspoon of extra-virgin olive oil

Directions

1. Preheat your oven to 450 degrees.
2. In a medium pot, combine the chicken broth and cauliflower florets. You may also use the stems as this makes a great stock for soups.
3. Season the pot carefully with a minimal amount of salt and pepper, following your doctor's orders.
4. Bring the pot to a boil and reduce to simmering.
5. Cover. Cook until the cauliflower is very tender – this should take approximately twenty minutes.
6. Puree the cauliflower until smooth. If you need to thin the cauliflower, use the broth.

THE TUNA SALAD

Serving Size: 2-3 tablespoons to ½ cup (Gradually increase after a few days)

Ingredients

1 can (6 oz.) Tuna packed in water, drained
1 tbsp. Pickle juice
1½ tbsp. Mayonnaise
1 tbsp. Powdered eggs

Directions

1. Combine ingredients in a blender and puree until smooth.

THE SHRIMP SPREAD

Serving Size: 2-3 tablespoons to ½ cup (Gradually increase after a few days)

Ingredients

1 pound cooked shrimp
¼ cup Hellmann's Reduced Fat mayonnaise
3 scallions chopped
1 teaspoon Old Bay Seasoning

Directions

1. Pulse shrimp in food processor until ground but still chunky. Transfer to bowl.
2. Place scallions, Mayonnaise, and Old Bay in food processor and pulse until scallions are very finely chopped.
3. Scrape flavoured mayonnaise to bowl with shrimp, and combine, adding a little water for desired texture.

THE PINTO BEAN DIP

Serving Size: 1- 2 tablespoons

Ingredients

1 small onion, diced
2 garlic cloves, chopped
2 teaspoons olive oil
One 15 ounce can pinto beans, drained and rinsed
1 cup of your favorite salsa
½ cup chicken broth

Directions

1. Sauté onion and garlic in olive oil in a non-stick skillet until golden brown.
2. Place beans, sautéed vegetables, and salsa to food processor and pulse until chunky, add broth a little at a time to desired consistency.
3. Pour mixture into skillet and cook until bubbly and thickened, about 10 minutes.

THE EGG SALAD

Serving Size: 2-3 tablespoons to 1/3 cup (Gradually increase after a few days)

Ingredients

4 hard-cooked eggs, chopped
2 tablespoons finely chopped green onion
2 tablespoons sliced Kalamata or black olives
¼ cup diced, seeded tomatoes
2 tablespoons reduced-fat mayonnaise
2 teaspoons milk
Salt and black pepper to taste
2 tbsps. crumbled feta cheese

Directions

1. Combine eggs, onion, olives and tomatoes.
2. Stir in mayonnaise, milk, and seasonings until well mixed.
3. Gently stir in cheese.
4. Place in a food processor and pulse until pureed.

CLASSIC HUMMUS

Serving Size: 2-3 tablespoons

Ingredients

1 clove garlic, smashed and peeled
1-15 ounce can chickpeas, rinsed
3 tablespoons fresh lemon juice
3 tablespoons extra-virgin olive oil
1 tablespoon tahini
1/2 teaspoon salt

Directions

1. In food processor, chop garlic until finely minced.
2. Scrape down the sides of food processor and add chickpeas, lemon juice, oil, tahini, and salt.
3. Process until completely smooth, scraping down sides as necessary (1-2 minutes).

THE AVOCADO SPREAD

Serving Size: 3-4 tablespoons

Ingredients

1 ripe, medium-sized avocado
2/3 cup white or cannellini beans, rinsed and drained
2 generous sprigs of cilantro
1 ½ tablespoons fresh lime juice (1-2 limes)
½ green jalapeno, seeds removed and chopped
½ teaspoon green Tabasco sauce
¼ teaspoon salt

Directions

1. In a blender or food processor blend all ingredients until smooth and creamy.

CREAMY CAULIFLOWER PUREE

Serving Size: 2-3 tablespoons to ¾ cup (Gradually increase after a few days)

Ingredients

1 large (6-7" diameter) head of cauliflower
3 cloves of garlic (cooked/steamed with cauliflower)
1/3 cup low-fat buttermilk
4 teaspoons extra-virgin olive oil
1 teaspoon butter, salted
½ teaspoon of garlic salt
½ teaspoon of black pepper

Directions

1. Break cauliflower into 2" x 2" pieces (or smaller) and put in large microwave safe bowl with ¼ cup water and 3 whole garlic cloves and cover.
2. Microwave for 5 minutes or until cauliflower is very tender.
3. Use garlic press to crush 3 garlic cloves and add them to food processor. Add cooked cauliflower to the food processor.
4. Add buttermilk, 2 teaspoons olive oil, butter, garlic salt, and pepper.
5. Process ingredients until smooth and creamy.
6. Drizzle the remaining 2 teaspoons of olive oil on top and serve.

Stage 4: Semi-Soft Foods

Yes, you may now move on to foodstuffs with a regular consistency, without fear. This is because your stomach is beginning to adapt to the new situation.

Acceptable foodstuffs include, but are not limited to low-fat dairy products, fruits, vegetables, whole grains, low-fat starches, fish, lean meat, pork and poultry. All of them are rich in essential nutrients.

Goals and Duration

This stage is expected to last for two weeks or even several months after your surgery.

At this time, when you are intent on consuming semi-soft foods only, you will be able to go back to three or five, well-balanced meals every day. These meals mainly comprise of solid foodstuffs, as well as ground or soft protein foods.

Of course, you will still have to consume the required amount of liquids throughout the day. They must take the place of snacks between meals.

The main aim is for you to recognize satiety when you feel it. Your earlier habit of overeating will be brought under control. As soon as you experience a feeling of satisfying fullness, you have to stop eating.

Diet Guidelines

Avoid foods that offer only empty calories, such as junk food, processed foods, etc. They are lacking in minerals, vitamins and proteins. This means that they are not nutrient-dense and therefore, can hardly be of any use to your body.

Since you can ingest only limited amounts of food at any given time, it is imperative that you go in for healthy meals. Eat the protein part first always.

Regardless of whatever menus you follow, you need extra supplements. Do not stop taking vitamin and mineral supplements at any cost.

Consume every meal slowly and patiently. Chew each chunk of food well, ensuring that the meal takes at least 20 to 30 minutes to complete. This will help in healthy digestion and absorption, as well as stretch the feeling of satiety for a longer time. You will automatically stop eating as soon as you feel full.

In case, you are still finding a large meal too difficult to handle, just go in for five or six small meals throughout the day.

You do not need to puree meat any longer. However, stay away from red meat for a few months, until the dietitian gives you permission to consume it. Whatever kind of meat dish you prepare, please ensure that you cut it into small portions before consuming it. Furthermore, do a good job of chewing every piece.

Bake, grill or broil your meats, since these are low-fat methods of cooking.

You can do away with protein shakes if your regular meals contain sufficient amounts of protein. Continue with them only if your requirements are not being met. For instance, women need at least 50 to 60 grams of protein each day, while men need around 60 to 70 grams every day. If you are still confused, consult your nutritionist.

With regard to vegetables, stay with cooked ones, and limit your consumption of raw ones. Season them with spices and herbs.

Eliminate raw broccoli stalks, corn and fresh asparagus from your diet.

Do not consume liquids at mealtimes. They may be consumed 30 minutes before, or 60 minutes after a meal.

It would be good to spread fluid intake over three hourly periods, which is, consuming half-a-cup every 30 minutes. This will take care of your fluid intake between meals.

Experiment with just one new food at a time.

Meal Suggestions

Protein Suggestions – You may try chopped lean meats, ham, lean ground Turkey, lean ground beef, Deli-sliced Turkey breast, roast beef, ham, chicken, shrimp, white fish, crab, lobster, tuna or chicken salad (with fat-free salad dressing or fat-free mayonnaise) and egg. Similarly, mashed or well-cooked black beans or pinto beans, low-fat cheese, tofu, poached eggs and hard-boiled eggs are good.

Grains and Starches – Well-cooked pasta, mashed or baked potatoes, low-fat crackers, toast, hot cereals and cereals soaked in milk, are good for your health.

Fruits and Vegetables – You may consume soft melon, bananas, canned pears or peaches (free of syrup), Mandarin oranges, plain berries (syrup-free and thawed after being frozen) and sugar-free applesauce. As for vegetables, you may opt for soft and well-cooked broccoli, carrots, beets, squash and green beans.

Sample Menu

Whenever you are eating a meal, you may opt for a main course like soft vegetables, combined with overcooked mashed potatoes, pasta or couscous.

The meal will taste even better if you add three-fourth tablespoons of scrambled eggs, fish in sauce or fish pie, baked beans, low-sugar cereal soaked in semi-skimmed or skimmed milk, macaroni cheese, cauliflower cheese, lasagna, Turkey or minced meat.

If you feel like snacking, go in for sugar-free custard, yoghurt, cottage cheese, rice pudding, sugar-free mousse, stewed fruit, soft tinned fruit, sugar-free whip or fromage frias.

Recipes: Stage 4

A MESSAGE FOR READERS

You must adjust the quantity of ingredients based on the servings you are preparing. The current quantities are generic and written to just give you an idea on which ingredient should be added in more quantity and which one in less quantity.

SEMI-SOLID FOODS RECIPES

Note: During this stage you can eat the recipes provided under Stage 3. The only change in preparation is to blend the food until semi-solid state than pureed. Below are three additional recipes provided that are good during Stage 4.

HEALTHY SCRAMBLED EGGS

Serving Size: 2-3 tablespoons to ½ cup (Gradually increase after a few days)

Ingredients

3 large egg whites
1 large egg yolk
2 tbsp. water
1/8 tsp. salt
1 tsp. unsalted butter
8 ounces fresh crimini mushrooms
Fresh ground black pepper

Directions

1. Place the egg whites, egg yolk, water and salt in a small mixing bowl and whisk until frothy.
2. Melt the butter in a small non-stick skillet pan over medium-high heat. Gently sauté the mushrooms until browned. Toss frequently. Cook the mushrooms until they are a dark caramel brown.
3. Add egg mixture and stir the eggs cooking until firm.
4. Add fresh ground black pepper to taste and serve.

MASHED CAULIFLOWER

Serving Size: 2-3 tablespoons to ½ cup (Gradually increase after a few days)

Ingredients

1 head of cauliflower
3 tablespoons milk
1 tablespoon low-fat butter
2 tablespoons light sour cream
1/4 teaspoon garlic salt
freshly ground black pepper
snipped chives

Directions

1. Separate the cauliflower into florets and chop the core finely.
2. Bring about 1 cup of water to a simmer in a pot, then add the cauliflower. Cover and turn the heat to medium. Cook the cauliflower for 12-15 minutes or until very tender.
3. Drain and discard all of the water (the drier the cauliflower is, the better) and add the milk, butter, sour cream, salt and pepper and mash with a masher until it looks like "mashed potatoes." Top with chives.

MASHED WHITE BEANS WITH GARLIC

Serving Size: 2-3 tablespoons to ½ cup (Gradually increase after a few days)

Ingredients

3 tablespoons olive oil
2 large cloves garlic, peeled, but left whole
1 sprig fresh rosemary
Two 14-ounce cans Cannellini beans, drained, rinsed
1-2 tablespoons chicken broth
1 tablespoon freshly grated Parmesan cheese
Kosher salt & black pepper
Olive oil

Directions

1. In a large skillet heat olive oil over medium-low heat.
2. Add whole garlic cloves and rosemary sprig. Sauté until garlic is soft and rosemary is crispy.
3. Smash garlic with the back of a wooden spoon. Remove rosemary, slide off the leaves and mince them; return to skillet.
4. Add beans and heat through, stirring and roughly mashing with the spoon, adding chicken broth until desired consistency.
5. Stir in Parmesan, salt, and black pepper.
6. Place in a serving bowl and drizzle with additional olive oil. Serve hot.

Stage 5: Regular Diet

Your Gastric Bypass surgery leads to alterations in hormone levels too. As a result, you may not feel inclined to eat much. In fact, you may even be tempted to skip meals, believing that this will hasten weight loss. Please do not indulge in such fantasies. You will find yourself becoming malnourished and weak. You may even experience hair loss. In order to avoid this, you must try to consume at least three plate-sized meals in a day, along with plenty of liquids.

Goals and Duration

This diet begins almost six weeks after your Gastric Bypass surgery. It is to be followed regularly thereafter.

The pureed stage is referred to as the stabilization diet. The semi-soft stage is akin to a maintenance diet. The regular stage is deemed as your diet for life.

By this time, you will be able to reach a firm conclusion about which foods agree very well with your "new" stomach. Then again, you will be able to tolerate some foods just moderately well. You may limit their consumption. Discard those foodstuffs from your list, which cause misery to your alimentary tract.

Whatever is the case, the aim is to ensure that your stomach obtains three or five, well-balanced meals every single day of your life. You may experiment with all kinds of recipes, provided all your meals are filled with essential nutrients.

Do not forget to include protein-rich foods in your menus. It is necessary to consume the protein portion first at every meal. This is to be followed by the consumption of carbohydrates, and then the rest.

Regardless of whatever you eat or drink, you are expected to take your required quota of vitamin and mineral supplements each day.

Finally, you are expected to adhere to the liquid diet also. Instead of snacking between meals, you must consume unflavored, calorie-free drinks.

Diet Guidelines

Despite crossing all the barriers successfully, you still need to be careful about ingesting unhealthy foodstuffs.

For instance, it would be advisable to avoid untoasted bread, stringy vegetables (spinach, celery and corn), seeds, nuts, coconut, tough meats, and vegetables or fruits with skins/membranes (potatoes, oranges, apples, grapefruit and pears). Do remember that you have not become immune to Dumping syndrome, constipation, diarrhea, blockages, etc.

Even if you were fond of alcohol prior to your Gastric Bypass surgery, avoid it altogether now. Spirits are high in calories. Some of them can even stimulate hunger pangs. As a result, you will end up overeating once again.

Even at this stage, it is imperative to remember that you cannot combine solid meals with fluids. If you wish to drink water or a no-calorie drink, do so at least half-an-hour before a meal. Alternatively, you may wait for an hour after the meal, before consuming liquids.

As far as liquids are concerned, you still need to consume 64 ounces every day. They are required to flush out the toxins from your digestive tract, keep you well hydrated and prevent constipation.

It would be good to consume liquids between meals, as they prevent unhealthy snacking. Furthermore, your stomach remains 'full.'

Experiment with just one novel food at any given time. Test your tolerance levels well before you continue with it.

Meal Suggestions

As some experts have suggested, you might keep the term FOG (farm, ocean and ground) in mind, when selecting foodstuffs for your regular diet.

For instance, products that have come from a farm are healthy. They include milk and other dairy products, eggs, Turkey and chicken are fresh and good.

Similarly, several kinds of fish, such as tuna, salmon, scallops, shrimp, Cod, etc. are suitable for your constitution.

Then again, vegetables, fruits, whole grains, etc. are grown in the ground. It would be better to adhere to cooked vegetables, rather than raw vegetables at this time. Later on, when your stomach feels more comfortable, you may try eating a few vegetables raw.

Here are some tips to bear in mind, when cooking your meals.

Baking, broiling, grilling or poaching is any day better than frying foodstuffs.

It is better to use vegetable or chicken broth, rather than oil. In fact, you may even use yoghurt or applesauce in recipes that call for a lot of oil or fat.

Lemon juice or spices make for better seasoning and flavoring agents, rather than butter or olive oil.

Sample Menu

Your breakfast may include half-a-cup or one-third cup of egg/yoghurt and half-a-cup of sugar-free fruit. Lunch could be a combination of one-fourth cup of sugar-free fruit, one-fourth cup vegetable and two ounces of meat (Turkey, fish, meat or chicken). Have the same for dinner too. Between meals, consume a cup of skimmed or 1% milk, as well as a cup of calorie-free drink/water. You can skip the milk at night. Drink only water.

Recipes: Stage 5

A MESSAGE FOR READERS

You must adjust the quantity of ingredients based on the servings you are preparing. The current quantities are generic and written to just give you an idea on which ingredient should be added in more quantity and which one in less quantity.

REGULAR DIET RECIPES

THE APPLE AND TUNA SANDWICHES

Serving Size: 1/3 of recipe

Ingredients

1 can tuna, packed in water (6.5 ounces, drained)
1 apple
¼ cup yogurt, low-fat vanilla
1 teaspoon mustard
½ teaspoon honey
6 slices whole wheat bread
3 lettuces leaves

Directions

1. Wash and peel the apple. Chop it into small pieces.
2. Drain the water from the can of tuna.
3. Put the tuna, apple, yogurt, mustard, and honey in a medium bowl. Stir well.
4. Spread ½ cup of the tuna mix onto each 3 slices of bread.
5. Top each sandwich with a washed lettuce leaf and a slice of bread.

THE COTTAGE CHEESE PANCAKES

Serving Size: 1 pancake

Ingredients

⅓ cup all-purpose flour
½ tsp. baking soda
1 cup low-fat cottage cheese
½ tablespoons canola oil
3 eggs, lightly beaten

Directions

1. Combine flour and baking soda in a small bowl.
2. Combine remaining ingredients in a large bowl.
3. Pour flour mixture into cottage cheese mixture and stir until just incorporated.
4. Heat a large skillet over medium heat, coat with cooking spray.
5. Pour ⅓ cup portions of batter onto skillet and cook until bubbles appear on the surface.
6. Flip and cook on the other side until brown.
7. Serve with low calorie syrup.

DEVILED EGGS

Serving Size: 2 deviled eggs

Ingredients

6 hard-boiled eggs (You will not use three of the yolks in this recipe.)
2 Tablespoons of creamy horseradish sauce or Greek yogurt
½ teaspoon dill
¼ teaspoon spicy mustard (Use Dijon for mild deviled eggs.)
⅛ teaspoon salt
Dash of black pepper and paprika

Directions

1. Peel the eggs and cut in half lengthwise.
2. Place 3 yolks into a mixing bowl, and set the whites aside. (Save the other three yolks for another use.)
3. Mash the yolks with creamy horseradish sauce or Greek yogurt, dill, mustard and salt.
4. Spoon or pipe filling into egg white halves.
5. Sprinkle with pepper and paprika.

BAKED TOMATOES

Serving Size: Two tomato halves

Ingredients

5-6 large tomatoes
Olive oil spray
¼ cup low fat parmesan cheese
Greek Seasoning (Penzey's is preferred)
¼ cup pine nuts (optional)

Directions

1. Preheat oven to 350 º F.
2. Cut tomatoes in half-lengthwise and place open face in non-stick 9x13 pan.
3. Spray surface of tomatoes with olive oil spray.
4. Coat with cheese and pine nuts.
5. Sprinkle on Greek seasoning to taste.
6. Bake for 50 minutes on middle rack.

COTTAGE CHEESE BAKE

Serving Size: 1/2 cup

Ingredients

2 cups low-fat or fat-free cottage cheese
2 whole eggs
10 oz. pack of frozen spinach (thawed and drained)
½ cup Parmesan cheese

Directions

1. Preheat oven to 350° F.
2. In large bowl, mix all ingredients together well.
3. Place evenly into 8x8 pan.
4. Bake for 20-30 minutes or until cheese bubbles on outside.
5. Let sit 5 minutes before serving.
6. Season to taste with salt, pepper, and garlic as desired.

THE CHICKEN CHEESESTEAK WRAP

Serving Size: 1 wrap

Ingredients

¼ pound boneless, skinless chicken breast, trimmed of visible fat
¼ cup onions, chopped
¼ cup green pepper, sliced
¼ cup mushrooms, sliced
1 wedge (¾ ounce) Laughing Cow Original light Swiss cheese or equivalent
1 whole wheat flour, low-carb tortilla
2 teaspoons sliced pickled hot chili peppers (optional)

Directions

1. Place chicken breast on cutting board, pound to 1/4" thin and slice into very thin strips.
2. Place a skillet over medium high heat and mist with cooking spray.
3. Add the onion and chicken to the heated pan and cook until onions are translucent and chicken is no longer pink throughout.
4. Add green peppers and mushrooms to the pan and cook until peppers and mushrooms soften.
5. Place tortilla between 2 damp paper towels. Microwave for 20 seconds.
6. Lay the warm tortilla flat and spread cheese in an even strip in the middle.
7. Top with chicken, peppers, onions and mushrooms.
8. Add chilli peppers if using.
9. Fold sides of tortilla over middle. Serve immediately.

THE EGG CHILADA

Serving Size: 1 egg-chilada

Ingredients

1 egg + 1 egg white
Black pepper and salt to taste
1 ounce protein of choice (tofu, chicken, or ground beef work well)
2 tablespoons salsa (such as Tostito's medium)
1 tablespoon shredded Mexican blend cheese
2 tablespoons plain fat-free Greek yogurt

Directions

1. Scramble the egg and egg white in a small bowl
2. Spray a skillet or griddle with cooking spray and set it over medium heat.
3. Pour the scrambled eggs onto the heated pan and allow it to spread into a generally circular shape.
4. Leave the eggs alone for a minute or two; allowing the edges to set. Add a sprinkle of black pepper and salt to the eggs while they're setting.
5. Slide a spatula beneath the eggs and flip (don't worry if some egg pours off at this point).
6. Cook eggs on the other side about two minutes or until completely cooked and transfer to a plate.
7. Make a strip of filling for your egg-chilada with 1 oz. protein of choice and Mexican cheese.
8. Roll up the egg "pancake" to form your egg-chilada.
9. Top with salsa and Greek yogurt.

CHICKEN IN GREEK YOGURT

Serving Size: 1 chicken breast

Ingredients

4 boneless skinless chicken breasts (4 oz. each)
1 cup plain Greek yogurt
½ cup grated Parmesan cheese
1 teaspoon garlic powder
1½ teaspoons seasoning salt
½ teaspoon pepper

Directions

1. Preheat oven to 375 degrees.
2. Combine Greek yogurt, cheese and seasonings in bowl.
3. Line baking sheet with foil and spray with cooking spray.
4. Coat each chicken breast in Greek yogurt mixture and place on foiled baking sheet.
5. Bake for 45 minutes.
6. Serve

PAN FRIED RAINBOW TROUT

Serving Size: 4 ounces

Ingredients

8 ounces rainbow trout fillets
3 tbsp. yellow cornmeal
1⅓ tbsp. chopped parsley
¼ tsp. ground celery seeds
¼ tsp. ground black pepper
1 pinch salt
2 tsp. olive oil

Directions

1. Clean and rinse fish fillets. Check to make sure all bones are removed. Pat dry.
2. Mix together cornmeal, salt, pepper, celery seed and chopped parsley.
3. Cover fish with cornmeal mixture and press onto fish.
4. Heat olive oil in non-stick skillet. Cook fish 2 to 3 minutes per side. Fish should be brown and crisp and should flake when pierced with a fork.

ASIAN PORK TENDERLOIN

Serving Size: 4 ounces

Ingredients

⅓ cup light soy sauce
⅓ cup brown sugar
2 tablespoons Worcestershire sauce
2 tablespoons lemon juice
2 tablespoons rice vinegar
1 tablespoon dry mustard
1 tablespoon ginger
1 ½ teaspoons pepper
4 garlic cloves or prepared minced
2 lbs. pork tenderloin

Directions

1. Mix ingredients together in freezer-safe bag.
2. Place tenderloin in freezer bag and rub marinade on pork.
3. Refrigerate overnight or place in freezer for future use.
4. Bake for 30-40 minutes at 375º F degrees OR prepare in slow cooker on low for 4-6 hours.

PORK AND BLACK BEAN STEW

Serving Size: 1/4 of recipe excluding rice

Ingredients

2 teaspoons extra-virgin olive oil
1 pound pork loin or tenderloin, trimmed of visible fat and cut into 1" cubes
1¼ cup chopped onions
3 cloves garlic
2 canned chipotle peppers in adobo sauce, minced plus 1 teaspoon adobo sauce
1 teaspoon ground cumin
1 packet Goya Sazon with coriander & annatto (or similar seasoning packet)
1 can (14 ounces) no salt added chicken broth
1 can (14.5 ounces) no salt added diced tomatoes in juice
1 can (14.5 ounces) no salt added black beans, drained & rinsed
1 teaspoon crushed red pepper flakes (optional)

Directions

1. In large pot or Dutch oven, heat olive oil over medium high heat.
2. Add pork cubes and cook, stirring occasionally for 4-6 minutes or until browned on all sides.
3. Add onion and garlic and cook for 2-3 minutes, or until starting to soften.
4. Add chipotle peppers and sauce, cumin, and seasoning packet. Stir to mix.
5. Add broth, tomatoes, beans and red pepper flakes if desired. Stir to mix well.

6. Bring stew to a boil then reduce heat to low.
7. Cover pot and simmer for 45 minutes to 1 hour, or until the port is fork tender.
8. Serve stew in bowls over brown rice or add rice to stew, if desired.

SWEET AND SOUR PORK

Serving Size: 1 cup of pork mixture and ½ cup of rice

Ingredients

Cooking spray
1 pound lean pork tenderloin, cut into thin strips
15 oz. canned, unsweetened pineapple chunks
½ cup water
¼ cup Splenda brown sugar blend
2 tbsp. corn starch
½ tsp. table salt
1 tbsp. low-sodium soy sauce
2 medium green peppers, sliced (as tolerated)
1 small onion, sliced (as tolerated)
3 cups cooked brown rice
1/3 cup wine vinegar

Directions

1. Heat a non-stick skillet coated with cooking spray over medium-high heat.
2. Add pork and cook until golden brown. Remove from skillet and set aside. Drain any remaining fat from skillet.
3. Drain pineapple chunks, reserving juice; set aside.
4. Combine water, vinegar, sugar, corn-starch, salt, soy sauce, and reserved pineapple juice in a small bowl. Add to skillet and cook until sauce is thickened, about 2 minutes.
5. Add pork to skillet and cook on low heat until meat is tender, stirring occasionally, for about 30 minutes.
6. Add peppers, onion, and pineapple chunks and cook for an additional 5 minutes. Serve over rice.

THE SLOW COOKER CHICKEN

Serving Size: 1 six-ounce portion

Ingredients

6 skinless, boneless chicken breasts (2 ½ lb.)
1 10 ¾ oz. reduced fat cream of mushroom soup
1 c. pureed cottage cheese or plain Greek yogurt
½ c. chicken stock
1 -.7 oz. envelope Italian dressing mix
1- 8 oz. pkg mushrooms
Cooking spray

Directions

1. Spray a large skillet with cooking spray. Cook chicken in batches over medium-high heat 2-3 minutes on each side or until just browned. Transfer chicken to a 5-qt. slow cooker.
2. Add soup, cottage cheese or yogurt, chicken stock, and Italian dressing mix to skillet. Cook over medium heat, stirring constantly, 2 to 3 minutes or until cheese is melted and mixture is smooth.
3. Arrange mushrooms over chicken in slow cooker. Spoon soup mixture over mushrooms. Cover and cook on LOW 4 hours. Stir well before serving.
4. To make ahead: Prepare recipe as directed. Transfer to a 13- x 9-inch baking dish, and let cool completely. Freeze up to one month. Thaw in refrigerator 8 to 24 hours. To reheat, cover tightly with aluminium foil, and bake at 325° for 45 minutes. Uncover and bake 15 minutes or until thoroughly heated.

SIMPLY FRIED RICE

Serving Size: ½ portion of the recipe

Ingredients

2 tablespoons low-sodium soy sauce
1 teaspoon mustard
1 teaspoon chili paste
1 teaspoon toasted sesame oil
3 ounces boneless, skinless chicken breast cut into ½" cubes
Black pepper, to taste
½ cup finely chopped whole green onions
¼ cup chopped carrot
1 clove garlic, minced
¾ cup cooked short-grain brown rice
¼ cup frozen peas
2 large egg whites
Olive oil spray

Directions

1. In a small bowl, combine soy sauce, mustard, chilli paste and sesame oil. Set aside.
2. Season the cubed chicken with black pepper.
3. Mist a large, non-stick wok or skillet with cooking spray and place over medium high heat until it is hot enough for a drop of water to sizzle on it.
4. Scatter the chicken cubes into the wok or skillet.
5. Cook, stirring occasionally, until browned on all sides and no longer pink inside.
6. Transfer chicken to a plate and cover to keep warm.
7. Lightly mist the wok or skillet with cooking spray again. Set

over medium-high heat.

8. Add the green onions, carrot, and garlic to the pan.
9. Cook, stirring frequently, for 2-3 minutes.
10. Add the cooked rice and peas.
11. Continue cooking and stirring for 2 minutes or until the mixture is hot throughout.
12. Using a spoon or spatula, create a hole in the rice and veggies to expose the center of the pan.
13. Off the heat, lightly mist the exposed part of the pan with cooking spray.
14. Add the egg whites and stir to mix them into the rice.
15. Cook for 1-2 minutes, or until the egg is completely cooked.
16. Return the chicken to the pan and stir in the reserved soy sauce mixture.
17. Leave on heat, stirring constantly, for about 1 minute or until heated. Serve immediately.

GINGER BEEF STIR FRY

Serving Size: 1/6 portion of the recipe

Ingredients

1 pound flank steak (cut into ¼-inch strips)
2 teaspoons ground ginger
2 medium garlic cloves
6 ounces beef broth (fat free)
¼ cup (2 ounces) hoisin sauce
3 tablespoons soy sauce
1 tablespoons cornstarch
1 teaspoon canola oil
¼ teaspoon crushed red pepper flakes
3 ounces broccoli florets
½ medium yellow, red or green bell pepper cut into strips
½ cup instant brown rice
2 medium stalks bok choy cut into ½-inch slices
8-ounce can sliced water chestnuts

Directions

1. In mixing bowl, stir together steak, garlic and ginger. Set aside.
2. Prepare rice according to directions on package.
3. Combine broth, hoisin sauce, soy sauce and corn-starch in a bowl. Stir until dissolved.
4. In wok or skillet, heat oil and red pepper flakes over medium-high heat.
5. Cook steak 4-5 minutes or until browned. Stir constantly. Set aside.
6. Put broccoli, bell pepper and carrot into pan. Cook over

medium-high heat for 2-3 minutes or until tender-crisp. Stir. (If mixture becomes too dry, add in 1-2 tablespoons water.)

7. Stir in bok choy and water chestnuts. Cook for additional 1-2 minutes or under bok choy is tender-crisp. Stir constantly.
8. Make a well in center of pan, and pour in broth.
9. Cook 1-2 minutes or until broth thickens, occasionally stir broth.
10. Mix in beef. Cook 1-2 minutes or until warm.
11. Serve over rice.

THE VEGETARIAN CHILI

Serving Size: 1 ½ cups

Ingredients

2 garlic cloves
2 teaspoons olive oil
1 large green bell pepper (diced)
1 cup onion chopped
½ lb. of sliced mushrooms
14.5 oz. can of diced tomatoes or 2 cups fresh tomatoes
8 oz. tomato sauce
2 tbsps. chili powder
1 medium zucchini (thinly sliced)
2- 15oz cans red kidney beans (rinsed)
10 oz. package of frozen corn
1 cup low fat shredded cheddar cheese

Directions

1. Heat olive oil and garlic in large pan.
2. Add onions, green pepper, and mushrooms. Cook until tender.
3. Add in tomato sauce, diced tomatoes, chilli powder, and bring to boil.
4. Turn down to low, add in zucchini and kidney beans. Simmer for 10-15 minutes.
5. Add frozen corn and ½ cup cheddar cheese. Stir.
6. Simmer on low for additional 10-15 minutes
7. Serve topped with cheddar cheese.

BROWN RICE AND BLACK BEAN CASSEROLE

Serving Size: 1/8 of recipe

Ingredients

1/3 cup brown rice
1 cup vegetable broth
1 tablespoon olive oil
1/3 cup diced onion
1 medium zucchini, thinly sliced
16 oz. cooked boneless, skinless chicken breast, chopped into small pieces
1/2 cup sliced mushrooms
1/2 teaspoon cumin
1/4 teaspoon cayenne pepper
1 (15 oz.) can black beans, drained
1 (4 oz.) can diced green chilies
1/3 cup shredded carrots
2 cups low fat Swiss cheese, shredded

Directions

1. Mix the rice and vegetable broth in a pot, and bring to a boil. Reduce heat to low, cover, and simmer 45 minutes or until rice is tender.
2. Preheat oven to 350° degrees F.
3. Lightly grease a large casserole dish with non-stick cooking spray.
4. Heat olive oil in skillet over medium heat, cook onion until

tender.

5. Mix in zucchini, chicken, mushrooms, and seasonings.
6. Cook and stir until zucchini is lightly browned and chicken is heated.
7. In large bowl, mix cooked rice, onion, zucchini, chicken, mushrooms, beans, chillies, carrots, and 1 cup Swiss cheese.
8. Transfer to prepared casserole dish and sprinkle with remaining 1 cup Swiss cheese.
9. Cover casserole loosely with foil, bake for 30 minutes in preheated oven.
10. Uncover, continue baking 10 minutes or until lightly browned.

THE PESTO

Serving Size: 1/2 cup

Ingredients

½ cup water
10oz package frozen, chopped spinach (thawed and well drained)
1/3 cup 1% cottage cheese
1/3 cup fresh basil (or 2 tbsp. dried basil) – fresh preferred
2 tbsps. grated parmesan cheese
1 tbsp. olive oil
2 cloves garlic, minced

Directions

1. Combine all ingredients in blender or food processor
2. Blend or process until smooth
3. Spoon ½ cup of mixture on poultry or fish

SQUASH AND APPLE BAKE

Serving Size: 1/6 of a pan

Ingredients

1 medium butternut squash, peeled & cut into ¾ inch cubes
2 medium apples, peeled, cored, and cut into thin wedges
1 tbsp. Splenda
1 tbsp. all-purpose flour
¼ cup melted butter
½ tsp. salt
2 tsps. ground cinnamon

Directions

1. Mix squash and apples together in a casserole dish.
2. Combine other ingredients and spoon over squash and apples and mix together.
3. Bake, covered, at 350 degrees F for 50-60 minutes, or until tender.
4. If you like a crispier topping, take lid off casserole dish for last 10 minutes of cooking

SMOOTH CHOCOLATE SOY DESSERT

Serving Size: ½ cup or 2-inch square

Ingredients

1 envelope unflavored gelatine
¼ cup hot water
1 package (1.4 oz.) sugar-free, fat-free chocolate fudge instant pudding
1 cup cold skim milk
16 ounces silken tofu
½ teaspoon vanilla extract
1 tablespoon cocoa powder (optional)
¼ teaspoon peppermint extract (optional)

Directions

1. In a small bowl, mix the hot water and unflavoured gelatine. Set aside and allow to firm.
2. In a medium-sized bowl, combine the cold skim milk and instant pudding mix.
3. Dice the tofu into ½- to 1-inch cubes and place in bowl with pudding mixture. Quickly whisk together to break up the soy cubes.
4. Add the vanilla extract and optional cocoa powder and peppermint extract.
5. Spoon the pudding and tofu mixture into a blender or food processor. Blend until smooth. You may need to blend for about 5 seconds and hand mix or shake the contents so that the motor does not stick.
6. Once the mixture has a smoothie-like texture, gradually add the gelatine until well combined and blend again.

7. Pour into a glass 8-inch dish, cover and place in refrigerator for at least 30 minutes to firm. The longer it sits, the firmer it will become.

8. Cut into eight portions and enjoy!

THE PUMPKIN MOUSSE

Serving Size: 1 cup

Ingredients

1 15oz can pumpkin
1 4oz package fat-free vanilla pudding
2 cups sugar-free whipped topping (i.e., Cool Whip)
½ cup skim milk
1 tsp. cinnamon
Allspice, nutmeg, ginger, clove and Splenda, to taste

Directions

1. Mix all ingredients together.
2. Whip until creamy smooth.

THE CHEESECAKE PUDDING

Serving Size: ¼ cup

Ingredients

1 cup plain fat-free Greek yogurt
1 package sugar-free cheesecake pudding mix

Directions

1.   Combine ingredients in a blender and puree until smooth.

Chapter 8

Dealing with Post Surgery Problems

Certain problems may crop up during the first few months following the operation.

Nausea and Vomiting

Even when you experience a sense of fullness in your stomach or excess pressure in your abdominal region, you refuse to stop eating. Hence, you vomit! It could also be that you are inclined towards rapid intake of foodstuffs or beverages. Other causes could be moving into the advanced diet stage too quickly, lack of proper chewing, consumption of hard-to-digest meats and other foods, drinking fluids along with meals, overeating, or lying down immediately after eating.

The best way to alleviate this problem is to chew small pieces of food thoroughly, before swallowing them. Eat and drink very slowly. Do not consume beverages with meals, but sip them slowly between meals. Stay away from processed foods filled with artificial sugars and large amounts of calories. Avoid fried, spicy, or greasy eatables. Rest your stomach by going back to a clear liquid diet for a couple of days.

Dumping Syndrome

Foodstuffs containing large amounts of carbohydrates or sugars cause abdominal cramping and pain, enhanced heart rate, diarrhea, nausea, sense of fullness, cold sweats, warmth and dizziness, since they cannot be digested by your new stomach. They are "dumped" into the small intestine, instead of being released slowly from the stomach. The symptoms show up within 15 minutes of your eating a meal.

The solution is simple. Just eliminate starchy, fatty and sugary foodstuffs from your diet.

Dehydration

This is a common occurrence, since you may not be consuming adequate amounts of liquids after your surgery. You may even be addicted to caffeine or alcohol.

Ensure that you consume at least 64 ounces (almost 2 liters) of fluids every day. You may sip them slowly throughout the day.

Pain in Chest and Shoulder

The culprit is your body positioning while the surgery is taking place. The blood has not been able to circulate properly and normally for quite some time, resulting in painful muscles. Even breathing and coughing may prove tiresome. This is the reason why nurses and physical therapists provide specific guidance.

With regard to breathing, take a deep breath first. Do not force the inhalation; be comfortable. Next, hold your breath for just a couple of seconds. Finally, release the air slowly and completely. Repeat the exercise thrice.

There is a method to coughing too. Inhale deeply, prior to coughing. Ensure that your cough comes up from the abdominal region, not the throat. A pillow held against the abdomen should provide adequate support. This exercise will help to loosen any secretions that may be lodged in your throat or lungs, thereby preventing pneumonia.

Do these exercises for your legs and feet, three times each. Stretch your toes towards the end of your bed, similar to pressing down upon a gas pedal. Pull them in, towards the head region of the bed. Relax. Circle each ankle to the right first, and then to the left. As for walking, cover short distances slowly.

Lactose Intolerance

If you experience bloating, flatulence, abdominal cramping and diarrhea as soon as you consume milk or other dairy products, you may have become lactose intolerant due to lactase enzyme deficiency caused by the surgery.

Seek professional advice to replace them with soymilk, Lactaid pills, or lactose-free milk.

Constipation

Since you are consuming lower quantities of food, fruits and vegetables, your bowel movements may become disturbed and rather irregular. At least, the frequency and volume may decrease in comparison to what they were like prior to surgery. In fact, you may experience emptying of bowels once in every three days. Constipation may also be associated with the usage of iron supplements.

Whatever is the case, you do not wish to have problems with intestinal blockages, hemorrhoids, or hernias later on, due to recurring constipation. Therefore, you may take recourse to over-the-counter laxatives like Citrucel or Metamucil; they are bulk forming. Actually, if you opt for high-fiber foods, consume plenty of sugar-free beverages and engage in regular physical activities, you may prevent constipation. If the problem is too severe, consult your PCP or Bariatric surgeon.

Diarrhea

Although rare in this kind of surgery, it is quite possible that your small intestine is not able to absorb digested food properly. Get it treated immediately. You might become dehydrated, otherwise. Other causes may be the consumption of antibiotics or lactose intolerance.

It would be best not to let this malady remain for long. Determine to limit your consumption of greasy, as well as high-fiber foods to the bare minimum. Do the same with milk and other dairy products. Stay away from fruits and vegetables, which are consumed with their skins intact. Similarly, avoid all caffeinated beverages and sugar alcohols. Ensure that you drink around 64 ounces (almost two liters) of fluids every single day.

Hair Loss

Probably, you are among the 10% or 20% of people, who experience thinning of hair after surgery. This process does not start immediately, but begins somewhere around three months later. Hair loss may continue for six months or so. This is because of protein and iron deficiencies in your diet.

Drinks containing protein supplements and iron supplements can help prevent hair loss. You have to ensure that your body obtains its quota of protein and iron requirements every day. Of course, the results your actions may not show up early; they may take time.

Vitamin and Mineral Deficiency

Decreased intake of food, malabsorption of digested food and reduction in the quantity of digestive juices, may lead to the deficiency of vitamin B12, folic acid, iron and calcium.

Since you have to place limitations on certain types of foods, it might be best to go in for supplements, instead. However, you will have to take these supplements as long as you live.

Food Intolerance

High-fiber foodstuffs, recipes that are high in fat content and foods that are difficult to chew are not welcomed by your new stomach. They include greens, pickles, tough meats, skins and seeds of vegetables and fruits, popcorn, highly spicy or seasoned foods, fried foods, bread and cereals prepared from whole grains, membranes of grapefruit and orange, stringy vegetables like string beans, asparagus and celery, fibrous vegetables, broccoli stalks, peas, beans, corn, dried fruits, coconut, granola and nuts. They tend to cause irritation, nausea and vomiting.

Try to stay away from the foods mentioned above, at least for six months after your surgery.

Heartburn

Known as gastro-esophageal reflux disease, it refers to the condition wherein the contents of the stomach, especially acids, are pushed back up into the esophagus. This results in a burning sensation in the chest region. It could be that you are addicted to pungent foods, overeating, or not consuming sufficient amounts of fluids. Then again, you probably had heartburn prior to the surgery itself.

Your physician may suggest antacids, since they tend to neutralize the acids in your stomach. Certain drugs either block or reduce the production of these acids. Do go in for a quick consultation, since the lining of the esophagus may be damaged due to these acids.

Bloating

The accumulation of excessive gas in your abdominal region may be due to the consumption of cruciferous vegetables (cauliflower, different types of cabbages, Brussels sprouts, broccoli and mustard greens), legumes, milk and milk products. Your stomach finds it difficult to digest them normally.

Apart from avoiding such foods and sugar alcohols for some time, you may request over-the-counter medications for releasing gas.

Blockage of Stomach Outlet

You need to remember that the Bariatric surgeon has narrowed the opening between your stomach and the small intestine during the operation. The aim is to prevent food from slipping into the small intestine too quickly, as well as to enhance the feeling of satiety. If you allow large pieces of bread, starchy foods, overcooked or chewy meat and nuts to enter your stomach, they will block this opening (anastomososis). Even large pills may be stuck.

Although these foodstuffs will dissolve on their own within a few hours, you will experience great discomfort until then. Try Pepto-Bismol. Switch over to soft foods like broth or gelatin for the next couple of days. In case, you experience food intolerance or chronic vomiting, consult your physician.

Stretching of Stomach Pouch

Keep filling your stomach to overflowing day after day, and you may find that it expands and ruptures.

If you wish to avoid this, learn to eat and drink as slowly as you can. Your stomach will experience a sense of fullness for a longer time, and prevent overeating. Do not snack between meals, but drink sugar-free beverages, instead. Liquids and solid food should never be combined during meals. Eat frequent meals, but consume smaller portions.

Gallstones

If you have gone into surgery with a BMI above 40, you may expect gallstones to show up after your surgery. This is because of your rapid weight loss.

The only option is to remove the gallbladder, because traditional methods of dissolving these stones or flushing them out may not work.

This Page Has Been Left Blank Intentionally.

Chapter 9

Supplements Suggestions

You are advised not to stop consuming vitamin and mineral supplements even after reaching your desired weight level. This is because you may become deficient in specific minerals and vitamins due to the ingestion of nutrient-depleted foodstuffs, lowered food intake and altered absorption. However, make sure that your supplements are in a liquid, chewable or crushable form, for large tablets and capsules may cause blockages. If their efficacy is not going to be affected, you may cut large tablets into smaller pieces, or even crush them completely.

Multivitamins with Minerals

You have two choices. Opt for the children's chewable multivitamins with iron or the adult Centrum chewable/liquid with iron. The former has to be consumed in alignment with the adult dosage prescribed on the label, while the latter has to be ingested once a day. Multivitamins will keep your body free of infections, as well as keep your nerves healthy. The mineral, iron will ensure that you do not become anemic.

Vitamin B12

If you wish your red blood cell count to remain normal and healthy, as well as your nervous system to function properly, you will need to add B12 to your dietary regimen. You may opt for oral consumption (500-mcg everyday) or injection (1000 mcg once a month).

Iron

This mineral has a very important role to play in your life. Several chemical processes, which occur within your body, receive an added impetus with the presence of iron. For instance, it ensures that oxygen reaches every cell in your body through your bloodstream. In case, your body cells failed to receive sufficient oxygen, you would feel extremely fatigued and incapable of reaching peak performance in whatever task you undertake. At the same time, you would become susceptible to all kinds of ailments, due to decreased immunity. Iron also regulates cell growth.

Do ensure that you consume 45 to 60 milligrams of iron daily.

Calcium and Vitamin D

Your bones, joints and teeth will remain healthy only if you consume sufficient calcium, along with vitamin D. Vitamin D ensures better absorption of calcium within your body. Therefore, the two are always taken in combination. You will need to take 1200 mg (two tablets of 600 mg each) daily.

B complex with Thiamine (B1)

All the carbohydrates that enter your body need to be converted into energy. Thiamine will take care of this, as well as ensure efficacious functioning of your nervous system, heart and muscles.

As the name suggests, B complex is a combination of several vitamins, which will help you to maintain healthy skin, hair, mouth, eyes and organs. Additionally, they will keep you energetic and emotionally stable.

Make sure that you take this combination supplement daily (1.5 mg).

Sample Schedule for Supplements

You may chart out your own schedule in alignment with your dietitian's instructions. The following sample is just meant to give you an idea.

If you take B12 and multivitamins with minerals in the morning, take calcium with vitamin D tablets at noontime and nighttime.

This Page Has Been Left Blank Intentionally.

Wrapping up!

Thanks to advancing medical knowledge and technological innovations, it has become possible for Bariatric surgeons to offer a viable solution regarding the problem of obesity and obesity-related diseases. The solution is Gastric Bypass surgery. Currently, four types of surgeries may be performed, in alignment with each patient's specifications. Of course, there is no denying that every kind of Gastric Bypass surgery, similar to several other surgeries, carries its own risks and complications.

However, you must realize that it is a lesser evil to face in comparison to suffering from chronic or life-threatening, obesity-related diseases all your life. In fact, this solution becomes more of a necessity rather than a matter of personal choice, if you have been fighting the battle of the bulge for years and years. You could have tried all kinds of weight-reduction programs and diets, but failed to achieve much success. Maybe, you could engage in some background research at the outset. Then, contact experienced professionals, consult people with a similar problem as yours and who have undergone Bariatric surgery, attend seminars, and so on, to gain some confidence.

When you feel that, you can move ahead without fear, request an appointment with a skilled Bariatric surgeon.

At last, I would like to thank you for reading this book and hope that you will create a new healthier you!

This Page Has Been Left Blank Intentionally.

RECIPES INDEX

STAGE 1: WATER   **28**

THE STRAWBERRY WATER   32
THE WATERMELON WATER   33
THE ORANGE & BLUEBERRY WATER   34
THE ROSEMARY & GRAPEFRUIT WATER   35
THE MANGO & GINGER WATER   36
THE MELON MIX WATER   37
SIMPLE CLEAR BEEF BONE BROTH   39
EASY CLEAR BEEF BONE BROTH - VERSION 2   40
SIMPLE CLEAR CHICKEN BONE BROTH   41
THE VEGETABLE BROTH   42

STAGE 2: SUGAR FREE CLEAR LIQUIDS   **44**

THE NERVE SOOTHER TEA   49
THE BRAIN GAINER TEA   50
THE GOOD MOOD TEA   51
LET'S FEEL LIGHT TEA   52
VITAMIN C BOOSTER TEA   53
GINGER & PEPPERMINT HERBAL TEA   54
THE EARL GREY HERBAL TEA   55
STRAWBERRY & LEMON HERBAL TEA   56
LOW-FAT CREAM OF MUSHROOM SOUP   58
LOW-FAT CREAM OF ASPARAGUS   60

STAGE 3: PUREED FOODS   **61**

PUREED BLACK BEAN SOUP   66
PUREED CAULIFLOWER SOUP   67
THE TUNA SALAD   68
THE SHRIMP SPREAD   69
THE PINTO BEAN DIP   70
THE EGG SALAD   71
CLASSIC HUMMUS   72
THE AVOCADO SPREAD   73
CREAMY CAULIFLOWER PUREE   74

STAGE 4: SEMI-SOFT FOODS   **75**

    HEALTHY SCRAMBLED EGGS   81
    MASHED CAULIFLOWER   82
    MASHED WHITE BEANS WITH GARLIC   83

STAGE 5: REGULAR DIET   **84**

    THE APPLE AND TUNA SANDWICHES   90
    THE COTTAGE CHEESE PANCAKES   91
    DEVILED EGGS   92
    BAKED TOMATOES   93
    COTTAGE CHEESE BAKE   94
    THE CHICKEN CHEESESTEAK WRAP   95
    THE EGG CHILADA   96
    CHICKEN IN GREEK YOGURT   97
    PAN FRIED RAINBOW TROUT   98
    ASIAN PORK TENDERLOIN   99
    PORK AND BLACK BEAN STEW   100
    SWEET AND SOUR PORK   102
    THE SLOW COOKER CHICKEN   103
    SIMPLY FRIED RICE   104
    GINGER BEEF STIR FRY   106
    THE VEGETARIAN CHILI   108
    BROWN RICE AND BLACK BEAN CASSEROLE   109
    THE PESTO   111
    SQUASH AND APPLE BAKE   112
    SMOOTH CHOCOLATE SOY DESSERT   113
    THE PUMPKIN MOUSSE   115
    THE CHEESECAKE PUDDING   116

Printed in Great Britain
by Amazon